Copyright ©2
RND

All rights reserved. No part of this publication may be reproduced, distributed, or transmitted in any form or by any means, including photocopying, recording, or other electronic or mechanical methods, without the prior written permission of the publisher, except in the case of brief quotations embodied in critical reviews and certain other noncommercial uses permitted by copyright law.

Table of Contents

Introduction 5
    What are the risk factors for fibromyalgia? 5
    Causes 6
    Who's affected 8
    Fibromyalgia symptoms 9
    Fibromyalgia fog | Fog 11
    Fibromyalgia symptoms in women | Symptoms in women .. 12
    Fibromyalgia in men 12
    Fibromyalgia trigger points 13
    Fibromyalgia pain 15
        Chest pain 15
        Back pain 16
        Leg pain 17
    Fibromyalgia causes 18
    Infections 19
    Genes 19
    Trauma 19
    Stress 20
    Fibromyalgia and autoimmunity 21
    Fibromyalgia risk factors 21
    Fibromyalgia diagnosis 23
    Fibromyalgia treatment 24

Fibromyalgia medication 25
   Antidepressants 26
   Antiseizure drugs 26
Fibromyalgia natural remedies 27
   Fibromyalgia diet recommendations 28
   Dietary strategies to keep in mind 29
   Fibromyalgia pain relief 30
   Living with fibromyalgia 32
   Fibromyalgia facts and statistics 33
   Self-help 34
      Exercise 35
      Aerobic exercise 36
      Resistance and strengthening exercises 37
      Pacing yourself 38
      Relaxation 39
   Better sleeping habits 40
   Fibromyalgia and diet 41
      Foods to include 43
      Foods to avoid 45
Fibromyalgia-friendly recipes 46
   Another study from BMC 52
   Focus on Vitamin D 53
   Say Yes to Fish 54

Foods to Avoid if You Have Fibromyalgia 54

Cut the Coffee and Processed Foods 55

Avoid Gluten and Limit Dairy 55

Keep an Eye on Additives 56

Say No to Nightshades 57

How to Create a Fibromyalgia Diet That's Right for You 58

Fibro-Friendly Snack Recipes 59

Simple Combo Snacks 62

Faux-Nut Snack 68

Introduction

Fibromyalgia (fi·bro·my·al·gi·a) is a condition that causes pain all over the body (also referred to as widespread pain), sleep problems, fatigue, and often emotional and mental distress. People with fibromyalgia may be more sensitive to pain than people without fibromyalgia. This is called abnormal pain perception processing. Fibromyalgia affects about 4 million US adults, about 2% of the adult population. The cause of fibromyalgia is not known, but it can be effectively treated and managed.

Fibromyalgia is a long-term (chronic) condition.

What are the risk factors for fibromyalgia?
Known risk factors include:

- Age. Fibromyalgia can affect people of all ages, including children. However, most people are diagnosed during middle age and you are more likely to have fibromyalgia as you get older.

- Lupus or Rheumatoid Arthritis. If you have lupus or rheumatoid arthritis (RA), you are more likely to develop fibromyalgia.
- Some other factors have been weakly associated with the onset of fibromyalgia, but more research is needed to see if they are real. These possible risk factors include:
- Sex. Women are twice as likely to have fibromyalgia as men.
- Stressful or traumatic events, such as car accidents, post-traumatic stress disorder (PTSD).
- Repetitive injuries. Injury from repetitive stress on a joint, such as frequent knee bending.
- Illness (such as viral infections).
- Family history.
- Obesity.

Causes
The exact cause of fibromyalgia is unknown, but it's thought to be related to abnormal levels of certain

chemicals in the brain and changes in the way the central nervous system (the brain, spinal cord and nerves) processes pain messages carried around the body.

It's also suggested that some people are more likely to develop fibromyalgia because of genes inherited from their parents.

It causes:

1. pain in the muscles and bones (musculoskeletal pain)
2. areas of tenderness
3. general fatigue
4. sleep and cognitive disturbances

This condition can be hard to understand, even for healthcare providers. Its symptoms mimic those of other conditions, and there aren't any real tests to confirm the diagnosis. As a result, fibromyalgia is often misdiagnosed.

In the past, some healthcare providers even questioned whether fibromyalgia was real. Today, it is much better understood. Some of the stigma that used to surround it has eased.

Fibromyalgia can still be challenging to treat. But medications, therapy, and lifestyle changes can help you to manage your symptoms and to improve your quality of life.

Who's affected
Anyone can develop fibromyalgia, although it affects around 7 times as many women as men.

The condition typically develops between the ages of 30 and 50, but can occur in people of any age, including children and the elderly.

It's not clear exactly how many people are affected by fibromyalgia, although research has suggested it could be a relatively common condition.

Some estimates suggest nearly 1 in 20 people may be affected by fibromyalgia to some degree.

One of the main reasons it's not clear how many people are affected is because fibromyalgia can be a difficult condition to diagnose.

There's no specific test for the condition, and the symptoms can be similar to a number of other conditions.

Fibromyalgia symptoms
Fibromyalgia causes what's now referred to as "regions of pain." Some of these regions overlap with what was previously referred to as areas of tenderness called "trigger points" or "tender points." However, some of these previously noted areas of tenderness have been excluded.

The pain in these regions feels like a consistent dull ache. Your healthcare provider will consider a diagnosis of fibromyalgia if you've experienced musculoskeletal pain in 4 out of the 5 regions of pain outlined in the 2016 revisions to the fibromyalgia diagnostic criteria.

This diagnostic protocol is referred to as "multisite pain." It's in contrast to the 1990 fibromyalgia diagnostic criteria definition for "chronic widespread pain."

This process of diagnosis focuses on the areas of musculoskeletal pain and severity of pain as opposed to an emphasis on pain duration, which was the previously the focal criteria for a fibromyalgia diagnosis.

Other symptoms of fibromyalgia include:

- fatigue
- trouble sleeping
- sleeping for long periods of time without feeling rested (nonrestorative sleep)
- headaches
- depression
- anxiety
- trouble focusing or paying attention
- pain or a dull ache in the lower belly
- dry eyes
- bladder problems, such as interstitial cystitis

In people with fibromyalgia, the brain and nerves may misinterpret or overreact to normal pain signals. This may be due to a chemical imbalance in the brain or abnormality in the dorsal root ganglionTrusted Source affecting central pain (brain) sensitization.

Fibromyalgia can also affect your emotions and energy level.

Fibromyalgia fog | Fog
Fibromyalgia fog – also known as "fibro fog" or "brain fog" – is a term some people use to describe the fuzzy feeling they get. Signs of fibro fog include:

- memory lapses
- difficulty concentrating
- trouble staying alert

According to a 2015 studyTrusted Source published in Rheumatology International, some people find mental fogginess from fibromyalgia more upsetting than pain.

Fibromyalgia symptoms in women | Symptoms in women
Fibromyalgia symptoms have generally been more severe in women than in men. Women have more widespread pain, IBS symptoms, and morning fatigue than men. Painful periods are also common.

However, when the 2016 revisions to the diagnostic criteria are applied, more men are being diagnosed with fibromyalgia, which may reduce the degree of distinction between the pain levels men and women experience. More research needs to be done to further evaluate that distinction.

The transition to menopause could make fibromyalgia worse.

Complicating things is the fact that some symptoms of menopause and fibromyalgia look almost identical.

Fibromyalgia in men
Men also get fibromyalgia. Yet, they may remain undiagnosed because this is seen as a woman's disease.

However, current statistics show that as the 2016 diagnostic protocol is more readily applied, more men are being diagnosed.

Men also have severe pain and emotional symptoms from fibromyalgia. The condition affects their quality of life, career, and relationships, according to a 2018 survey published in the American Journal of Public Health.

Part of the stigma and difficulty in getting diagnosed stems from society's expectation that men who are in pain should "suck it up."

Men who do venture in to see a doctor can face embarrassment, and the chance that their complaints won't be taken seriously.

Fibromyalgia trigger points
In the past, people were diagnosed with fibromyalgia if they had widespread pain and tenderness in at least 11 out of 18 specific trigger points around their body.

Healthcare providers would check to see how many of these points were painful by pressing firmly on them.

Common trigger points included the:

- back of the head
- tops of the shoulders
- upper chest
- hips
- knees
- outer elbows

For the most part, trigger points are no longer a part of the diagnostic process.

Instead, healthcare providers may diagnose fibromyalgia if you've had pain in 4 out of the 5 areas of pain as defined by the 2016 revised diagnostic criteria, and you have no other diagnosable medical condition that could explain the pain.

Fibromyalgia pain
Pain is the hallmark fibromyalgia symptom. You'll feel it in various muscles and other soft tissues around your body.

The pain can range from a mild achiness to an intense and almost unbearable discomfort. Its severity could dictate how well you cope day to day.

Fibromyalgia appears to stem from an abnormal nervous system response. Your body overreacts to things that shouldn't normally be painful. And you may feel the pain in more than one area of your body.

However, available research still doesn't pinpoint an exact cause for fibromyalgia. Research continues to evolve in better understanding this condition and its origin.

Chest pain
When fibromyalgia pain is in your chest, it can feel frighteningly similar to the pain of a heart attack.

Chest pain in fibromyalgia is actually centered in the cartilage that connects your ribs to your breastbone. The pain may radiate to your shoulders and arms.

Fibromyalgia chest pain may feel:

- sharp
- stabbing
- like a burning sensation

And similar to a heart attack, it can make you struggle to catch your breath.

Back pain
Your back is one of the most common places to feel pain. About 80 percent of Americans have low back pain at some point in their lives. If your back hurts, it may not be clear whether fibromyalgia is to blame, or another condition like arthritis or a pulled muscle.

Other symptoms like brain fog and fatigue can help pinpoint fibromyalgia as the cause. It's also possible to have a combination of fibromyalgia and arthritis.

The same medications you take to relieve your other fibromyalgia symptoms can also help with back pain. Stretching and strengthening exercises can help provide support to the muscles and other soft tissues of your back.

Leg pain
You can also feel fibromyalgia pain in the muscles and soft tissues of your legs. Leg pain can feel similar to the soreness of a pulled muscle or the stiffness of arthritis. It can be:

- deep
- burning
- throbbing

Sometimes fibromyalgia in the legs feels like numbness or tingling. You may have a creepy crawling sensation.

An uncontrollable urge to move your legs is a sign of restless legs syndrome (RLS), which can overlap with fibromyalgia.

Fatigue sometimes manifests in the legs. Your limbs can feel heavy, as if they're held down by weights.

Fibromyalgia causes
Healthcare providers and researchers don't know what causes fibromyalgia.

According to the latest research, the cause appears to be a multiple-hit theory that involves genetic disposition (hereditary characteristics) complemented by a trigger, or a set of triggers, such as infection, trauma, and stress.

Let's take a closer look at these potential factors and several more that may influence why people develop fibromyalgia.

Infections
A past illness could trigger fibromyalgia or make its symptoms worse. The flu, pneumonia, GI infections, such as those caused by Salmonella and Shigella bacteria, and the Epstein-Barr virus all have possible links to fibromyalgia.

Genes
Fibromyalgia often runs in families. If you have a family member with this condition, you're at higher risk for developing it.

Researchers think certain gene mutations may play a role. They've identified a few possible genes that affect the transmission of chemical pain signals between nerve cells.

Trauma
People who go through a severe physical or emotional trauma may develop fibromyalgia. The condition has

been linkedTrusted Source to post-traumatic stress disorder (PTSD).

Stress

Like trauma, stress can leave long-lasting effects on your body. Stress has been linked to hormonal changes that could contribute to fibromyalgia.

Healthcare providers don't fully understand what causes the chronic widespread nature of fibromyalgia pain. One theory is that the brain lowers the pain threshold. Sensations that weren't painful before become very painful over time.

Another theory is that the nerves overreact to pain signals.

They become more sensitive, to the point where they cause unnecessary or exaggerated pain.

Fibromyalgia and autoimmunity

In autoimmune diseases like rheumatoid arthritis (RA) or multiple sclerosis (MS), the body mistakenly targets its own tissues with proteins called autoantibodies. Just like it would normally attack viruses or bacteria, the immune system instead attacks the joints or other healthy tissues.

Fibromyalgia symptoms look very similar to those of autoimmune disorders. These symptom overlaps have led to the theory that fibromyalgia could be an autoimmune condition.

This claim has been hard to prove, in part because fibromyalgia doesn't cause inflammation, and to-date reproducing autoantibodies haven't been found.

Yet, it's possible to have an autoimmune disease and fibromyalgia simultaneously.

Fibromyalgia risk factors
Fibromyalgia flare-ups can be the result of:

- stress

- injury
- an illness, such as the flu

An imbalance in brain chemicals may cause the brain and nervous system to misinterpret or overreact to normal pain signals.

Other factors that increase your risk of developing fibromyalgia include:

Gender. Most fibromyalgia cases are currently diagnosed in women, although the reason for this gender disparity isn't clear.

Age. You're most likely to be diagnosed in middle age, and your risk increases as you get older. However, children can develop fibromyalgia also.

Family history. If you have close family members with fibromyalgia, you may be at greater risk for developing it.

Disease. Although fibromyalgia isn't a form of arthritis, having lupus or RA may increase your risk of also having fibromyalgia.

Fibromyalgia diagnosis

Your healthcare provider may diagnose you with fibromyalgia if you've had widespread pain for 3 months or longer. "Widespread" means the pain is on both sides of your body, and you feel it above and below your waist.

After a thorough examination, your healthcare provider must conclude that no other condition is causing your pain.

No lab test or imaging scan can detect fibromyalgia. Your healthcare provider may use these tests to help rule out other possible causes of your chronic pain.

Fibromyalgia can be hard for healthcare providers to distinguish from autoimmune diseases because the symptoms often overlap.

Some research has pointed to a link between fibromyalgia and autoimmune diseases like Sjogren's syndrome.

Fibromyalgia treatment
Currently, there isn't a cure for fibromyalgia.

Instead, treatment focuses on reducing symptoms and improving quality of life with:

- medications
- self-care strategies
- lifestyle changes

Medications can relieve pain and help you sleep better. Physical and occupational therapy improve your strength and reduce stress on your body. Exercise and stress-reduction techniques can help you feel better, both mentally and physically.

In addition, you may wish to seek out support and guidance. This may involve seeing a therapist or joining a support group.

In a support group, you can get advice from other people who have fibromyalgia to help you through your own journey.

Fibromyalgia medication

The goal of fibromyalgia treatment is to manage pain and improve quality of life. This is often accomplished through a two-pronged approach of self-care and medication.

Common medications for fibromyalgia include:

- Pain relievers
- Over-the-counter pain relievers such as ibuprofen (Advil) or acetaminophen (Tylenol) can help with mild pain.
- Narcotics, such as tramadol (Ultram), which is an opioid, were previously prescribed for pain relief. However, research has shown they're not effective. Also, the dosage for narcotics is typically increased rapidly, which can pose a health risk for those prescribed these drugs.

Most healthcare providers recommend avoiding narcotics to treat fibromyalgia.

Antidepressants
Antidepressants such as duloxetine (Cymbalta) and milnacipran HCL (Savella) are sometimes used to treat pain and fatigue from fibromyalgia. These medications may also help improve sleep quality and work on rebalancing neurotransmitters.

Antiseizure drugs
Gabapentin (Neurontin) was designed to treat epilepsy, but it may also help reduce symptoms in people with fibromyalgia. Pregabalin (Lyrica), another anti-seizure drug, was the first drug FDA-approved for fibromyalgia. It blocks nerve cells from sending out pain signals.

A few drugs that aren't FDA-approved to treat fibromyalgia, including antidepressants and sleep aids, can help with symptoms. Muscle relaxants, which were once used, are no longer recommended.

Researchers are also investigating a few experimental treatments that may help people with fibromyalgia in the future.

Fibromyalgia natural remedies

If the medications your healthcare provider prescribes don't entirely relieve your fibromyalgia symptoms, you can look for alternatives. Many natural treatments focus on lowering stress and reducing pain. You can use them alone or together with traditional medical treatments.

Natural remedies for fibromyalgia include:

- physical therapy
- acupuncture
- 5-hydroxytryptophan (5-HTP)
- meditation
- yoga, use with caution if hypermobility is present
- tai chi
- exercise
- massage therapy

- a balanced, healthy diet

Therapy can potentially reduce the stress that triggers fibromyalgia symptoms and depression.

Group therapy may be the most affordable option, and it will give you a chance to meet others who are going through the same issues.

Cognitive behavioral therapy (CBT) is another option that can help you manage stressful situations. Individual therapy is also available if you prefer one-on-one help.

It's important to note that most alternative treatments for fibromyalgia haven't been thoroughly studied or proven effective.

Ask your healthcare provider about the benefits and risks before trying any of these treatments.

Fibromyalgia diet recommendations
Some people report that they feel better when they follow a specific diet plan or avoid certain foods. But

research hasn't proven that any one diet improves fibromyalgia symptoms.

If you've been diagnosed with fibromyalgia, try to eat a balanced diet overall. Nutrition is important in helping you to keep your body healthy, to prevent symptoms from getting worse, and to provide you with a constant energy supply.

Dietary strategies to keep in mind:

- Eat fruits and vegetables, along with whole grains, low-fat dairy, and lean protein.
- Drink plenty of water.
- Eat more plants than meat.
- Reduce the amount of sugar in your diet.
- Exercise as often as you can.
- Work toward achieving and maintaining your healthy weight.

You may find that certain foods make your symptoms worse, such as gluten or MSG. If that's the case, keep a food diaryTrusted Source where you track what you eat and how you feel after each meal.

Share this diary with your healthcare provider. They can help you identify any foods that aggravate your symptoms. Avoiding these foods can be beneficial helping you manage your symptoms.

Fibromyalgia can leave you feeling tired and worn out.

A few foods will give you the energy boost you need to get through your day.

Fibromyalgia pain relief
Fibromyalgia pain can be uncomfortable and consistent enough to interfere with your daily routine. Don't just settle for pain. Talk to your healthcare provider about ways to manage it.

One option is to take pain relievers such as:

- aspirin
- ibuprofen

- naproxen sodium
- help with discomfort
- lower pain levels
- help you better manage your condition

These medications bring down inflammation. Though inflammation is not a primary part of fibromyalgia, it may be present as an overlap with RA or another condition. Pain relievers may help you sleep better.

Please note that NSAIDS do have side effects. Caution is advised if NSAIDS are used for an extended period of time as is usually the case in managing a chronic pain condition.

Talk with your healthcare provider to create a safe treatment plan that works well in helping you manage your condition.

Antidepressants and anti-seizure drugs are two other medication classes your healthcare provider may prescribe to manage your pain.

The most effective pain reliever does not come in a medication bottle.

Practices like yoga, acupuncture, and physical therapy can:

- Fibromyalgia fatigue can be just as challenging to manage as pain.
- Learn a few strategies to help you sleep better and feel more alert during the day.

Living with fibromyalgia
Your quality of life can be affected when you live with pain, fatigue, and other symptoms on a daily basis. Complicating things are the misunderstandings many people have about fibromyalgia. Because your symptoms are hard to see, it's easy for those around you to dismiss your pain as imaginary.

Know that your condition is real. Be persistent in your pursuit of a treatment that works for you. You may need to try more than one therapy, or use a few techniques in combination, before you start to feel better.

Lean on people who understand what you're going through, like:

- your healthcare provider
- close friends
- a therapist

Be gentle on yourself. Try not to overdo it. Most importantly, have faith that you can learn to cope with and manage your condition.

Fibromyalgia facts and statistics
Fibromyalgia is a chronic condition that causes:

- widespread pain
- fatigue
- difficulty sleeping
- depression

Currently, there's no cure, and researchers don't fully understand what causes it. Treatment focuses on medications and lifestyle changes to help ease the symptoms.

About 4 million AmericansTrusted Source ages 18 and over, or about 2 percent of the population, have been diagnosed with fibromyalgia. Most fibromyalgia cases are diagnosed in women, but men and children can also be affected.

Most people get diagnosed in middle age.

Fibromyalgia is a chronic (long-term) condition. However, some people may experience remission-type periods in which their pain and fatigue improve.

Self-help
If you have fibromyalgia, there are several ways to change your lifestyle to help relieve your symptoms and make your condition easier to live with.

Your GP, or another healthcare professional treating you, can offer advice and support about making these changes part of your everyday life.

There are organisations to support people with fibromyalgia that may also be able to offer advice.

Exercise
As extreme tiredness (fatigue) and pain are 2 of the main symptoms of fibromyalgia, you may find that you're not able to exercise as much as you'd like.

But an exercise programme specially suited to your condition can help you manage your symptoms and improve your overall health.

Your GP or physiotherapist may be able to refer you to a health professional who specialises in helping people with fibromyalgia work out an exercise plan.

The plan is likely to involve a mixture of aerobic and strengthening exercises.

Aerobic exercise
Aerobic activities are any kind of rhythmic, moderate-intensity exercises that increase your heart rate and make you breathe harder.

Examples include:

- walking
- cycling
- swimming

Research suggests that aerobic fitness exercises should be included in your personalised exercise plan, even if you cannot complete these at a high level of intensity.

For example, if you find jogging too difficult, you could try brisk walking instead.

A review of a number of studies found aerobic exercises may improve quality of life and relieve pain.

As aerobic exercises increase your endurance (how long you can keep going), these may also help you function better on a day-to-day basis.

Resistance and strengthening exercises

Resistance and strengthening exercises are those that focus on strength training, such as lifting weights.

These exercises need to be planned as part of a personalised exercise programme. If they're not, muscle stiffness and soreness could be made worse.

A review of a number of studies concluded that strengthening exercises may improve:

- muscle strength
- physical disability
- depression
- quality of life

People with fibromyalgia who completed the strengthening exercises in these studies said they felt less tired, could function better and experienced a boost in mood.

Improving the strength of your major muscle groups can make it easier to do aerobic exercises.

Pacing yourself
If you have fibromyalgia, it's important to pace yourself. This means balancing periods of activity with periods of rest, and not overdoing it or pushing yourself beyond your limits.

If you do not pace yourself, it could slow down your progress in the long term.

Over time, you can gradually increase your periods of activity while making sure they're balanced with periods of rest.

If you have fibromyalgia, you'll probably have some days when your symptoms are better than others.

Try to maintain a steady level of activity without overdoing it, but listen to your body and rest whenever you need to.

Avoid any exercise or activity that pushes you too hard as this can make your symptoms worse.

If you pace your activities at a level that's right for you, rather than trying to do as much as possible in a short space of time, you should make steady progress.

For example, it may help to start with gentler forms of exercise, such as tai chi, yoga and pilates, before attempting more strenuous aerobic or strengthening exercises.

Relaxation
If you have fibromyalgia, it's important to regularly take time to relax or practise relaxation techniques.

Stress can make your symptoms worse or cause them to flare up more often. It could also increase your chances of developing depression.

There are many relaxation aids available, including books, tapes and courses, although deep-breathing techniques or meditation may be just as effective.

Try to find time each day to do something that relaxes you. Taking time to relax before bed may also help you sleep better at night.

Talking therapies, such as counselling, can also be helpful in combating stress and learning to deal with it effectively.

Your GP may recommend you try this as part of your treatment.

Better sleeping habits
Fibromyalgia can make it difficult to fall asleep or stay asleep, known as insomnia.

If you have problems sleeping, it may help to:

- get up at the same time every morning
- try to relax before going to bed
- try to create a bedtime routine, such as taking a bath and drinking a warm, milky drink every night

- avoid caffeine, nicotine and alcohol before going to bed
- avoid eating a heavy meal late at night
- make sure your bedroom is a comfortable temperature and is quiet and dark
- avoid checking the time throughout the night

Fibromyalgia and diet

Fibromyalgia is a chronic condition that's characterized by widespread muscle pain. Due to chronic pain, many people with fibromyalgia also have sleep disorders, chronic fatigue, and depression.

The cause of fibromyalgia isn't yet known, and the condition cannot be cured. People with fibromyalgia must manage their symptoms through medical treatment and lifestyle changes.

One way to help symptoms is by following a certain diet.

Though little research has been done, some evidence points to certain dietary approaches that may help manage fibromyalgia symptoms. These include:

Low calorie diets. Weight loss may help with fibromyalgia symptoms, so a low calorie diet may be a good approach.

Vegetarian diets. These diets are rich in anti-inflammatory fruits, vegetables, nuts, and legumes. The strongest evidence is for raw vegetarian diets.

Low FODMAP diets. FODMAPS are types of carbs that some people can't digest. Low FODMAP diets exclude most dairy products, grains, fruits, and vegetables. It's a very restrictive, highly anti-inflammatory way of eating.

A diet high in anti-inflammatory foods may also help manage fibromyalgia symptoms, as chronic inflammation is one of the suspected causes of the disease.

Regardless, this disease and its symptoms are highly individualized. Different diets may work better or worse depending on the individual.

You may benefit from working with a registered dietitian if you're following a more complex eating pattern, such as a raw vegetarian or low FODMAP diet, to manage your fibromyalgia symptoms.

Foods to include
Types of foods that are typically part of dietary approaches for fibromyalgia include:

- Low calorie: low calorie, high protein, high fiber, or filling foods like fruits, vegetables, lean proteins, and whole grains
- Vegetarian: fruits, vegetables, legumes, nuts, and seeds; some vegetarians may include eggs or dairy products while raw vegetarians eat only uncooked plant foods

- Low FODMAP: only foods that are low in FODMAPs, including most meats, rice, some fruits and vegetables, and limited dairy products
- You should also add a variety of anti-inflammatory foods that fit into your preferred eating pattern, as they may help alleviate symptoms. Examples of anti-inflammatory foods include:
- Protein: salmon, eggs, chickpeas, Greek yogurt
- Fruits: bananas, oranges, apples, grapes, blueberries, strawberries, blackberries, tomatoes, avocado
- Vegetables: spinach, kale, zucchini, cauliflower, broccoli, cabbage, bell peppers, cucumber, carrots
- Carbs: sweet potatoes, brown rice, honey
- Fats: olive oil, coconut oil
- Herbs and spices: turmeric, ginger, cinnamon, rosemary, garlic, cloves

Note that some of these foods, such as honey and chickpeas, are higher in FODMAPs. As such, avoid them if you're strictly following a low FODMAP diet.

Foods to avoid

On the other hand, foods that are typically avoided in the dietary approaches to fibromyalgia are:

- Low calorie. Exclude empty calories like chips, cookies, cakes, ice cream, sugary drinks, added sugars, and added fats.
- Vegetarian. All vegetarians exclude meat from their diet. However, raw vegetarians will also exclude cooked foods.
- Low FODMAP. On the low FODMAP diet, you need to exclude all foods that are high in FODMAPs. This includes wheat, dairy products, beans, garlic, and onions.

Anti-inflammatory. To decrease inflammation you should also avoid pro-inflammatory foods, which include highly processed foods, refined carbs, fast food, and processed vegetable oils like soybean oil or corn oil.

Fibromyalgia-friendly recipes

The following recipes are appropriate for various dietary approaches to fibromyalgia, and they all contain anti-inflammatory ingredients like fruits, vegetables, herbs, and spices.

1. Shakshuka for one (vegetarian, low FODMAP)

Shakshuka is a North African dish made by simmering eggs in tomato sauce. However, this take includes some healthy, anti-inflammatory additions like spinach and fresh parsley.

At only 286 calories per serving, it's also an ideal meal for anyone following a low calorie diet to help manage their fibromyalgia.

It's likewise appropriate for anyone following a lacto-ovo-vegetarian diet, which includes eggs and dairy products.

Simply swap the onions and garlic for garlic- and/or shallot-infused olive oil to make it FODMAP-free.

2. Mango turmeric overnight oats (vegetarian)

This easy breakfast dish is appropriate for raw vegetarian diets, as you don't have to cook it. Instead, the oats soften overnight by soaking in coconut milk, resulting in a creamy and smooth texture.

Additionally, this recipe contains several anti-inflammatory ingredients like ginger, cinnamon, turmeric, and honey.

3. Watermelon, mint, and grilled cheese salad (vegetarian)

This flavorful salad makes a great summer meal. With 484 calories in a generous serving, it can be part of a carefully planned low calorie diet.

It's also appropriate for lacto-vegetarian diets, which include dairy products.

Finally, the salad is rich in vitamin C — a potent anti-inflammatory antioxidant — from the watermelon.

4. Wild blueberry cauliflower smoothie (vegetarian)

Smoothies are a perfect on-the-go meal solution, and this vegan smoothie is compatible with a raw vegetarian diet for fibromyalgia. Because it contains only 340 calories per serving, it's also an appropriate meal for low calorie diets.

It contains blueberries, strawberries, and purple cauliflower, which are all rich sources of anthocyanins — antioxidant pigments that give these fruits and vegetables their bright colors.

Anthocyanins are also highly anti-inflammatory, with one study showing they improved sleep quality in people with fibromyalgia. However, more research is needed

5. Mediterranean vegetable salad with prunes and fruit dressing (vegetarian)

This vegan salad recipe is loaded with anti-inflammatory ingredients like prunes and beets.

With a few simple tweaks, like opting to not cook down the prune juice and swapping out the edamame for nuts like walnuts or pecans, you can make this a raw vegan recipe.

Additionally, this entrée salad contains only 450 calories in a large portion — making it a good fit for a low calorie diet.

6. Fresh spring rolls (vegetarian, low FODMAP)

These low FODMAP spring rolls are loaded with vegetables and are naturally low in calories — containing only 240 calories in a 3-roll serving.

They're also full of a variety of antioxidants from colorful vegetables like carrots, zucchini, bell pepper, and red cabbage.

For an extra dose of protein, you can add tofu or cooked shrimp.

7. Chocolate mint quinoa breakfast bowl (vegetarian, low FODMAP)

This indulgent breakfast recipe is loaded with antioxidants from anti-inflammatory berries, dark chocolate, and pumpkin seeds.

At 490 calories per serving, it's a bit high in calories for breakfast on a low calorie diet. However, you could easily include a smaller portion of this breakfast bowl or split it into two meals.

It's also vegetarian and low in FODMAPs, making it ideal for people with fibromyalgia.

8. Trail mix (vegetarian, low FODMAP)

This quick and easy trail mix recipe is a perfect vegetarian and low FODMAP grab-and-go snack. It can fit into a low calorie diet as well, as it only contains 140 calories per serving.

It contains antioxidant-rich pecans, pumpkin seeds, bananas, and dark chocolate — which may help decrease chronic inflammation.

9. Sprouted rice salad (vegetarian, low FODMAP)

This salad can be eaten warm or cold, so it's a great vegetarian and low FODMAP dinner or lunch option. It also contains only 280 calories per serving, making it a good choice for low calorie diets as well.

It's rich in anti-inflammatory antioxidants from pomegranate, including vitamin C

10. Low carb chicken salad on zucchini chips (low FODMAP)

This low FODMAP chicken salad can easily be made vegetarian by replacing the chicken with hard-boiled eggs or cubed tofu.

It's full of anti-inflammatory ingredients, like grapes, pecans, purple cabbage, and rosemary.

At only 265 calories per serving, it can also be eaten on a low calorie diet.

Another study from BMC
Complementary Alternative Medicine had similar findings. It concluded that fibromyalgia symptoms may be relieved by a mostly raw, vegetarian diet.

You don't have to go all-out vegan or strictly vegetarian, but aim to eat plenty of fresh fruits and vegetables to ensure you get a wide array of important antioxidants. Plus, eating fresh fruits and veggies, as opposed to processed foods full of potentially irritating preservatives, can help improve irritable bowel syndrome (IBS) symptoms. Similarly, you may want to opt for organic produce when possible to avoid consuming pesticides that may trigger pain.

Focus on Vitamin D
A vitamin D deficiency can cause muscle weakness and bone pain, which may make symptoms of fibromyalgia worse. Ask your doctor to check your vitamin D status regularly, and discuss a supplement if your levels are below optimum.

It's also a good idea to eat vitamin D-rich foods daily. Vitamin D can be found in fatty fish, eggs, and fortified products like cereal, milk and orange juice.

According to a study in the journal Pain, people who have higher vitamin D levels may experience less pain than people with lower levels. In the study, 30 women living with fibromyalgia were divided between two groups: one that took a placebo medication and one that received oral vitamin D supplements. After six months, the group that had received vitamin D reported feeling less pain than the placebo group. This was a small study, however, so more research is needed.

Say Yes to Fish
Omega-3 fatty acids are lauded for their ability to improve heart health and reduce inflammation, and it's thought that this nutrient could also help reduce stiffness and soreness in people with fibromyalgia. You can find this healthy fat in certain fish like salmon, as well as some nuts and seeds.

Foods to Avoid if You Have Fibromyalgia
In a study published in Clinical Rheumatology, 42 percent of the 65 patients with fibromyalgia surveyed said their symptoms were aggravated after eating certain foods. Avoiding some foods may help you reduce symptoms of fibromyalgia or prevent them altogether.

Cut the Coffee and Processed Foods
Though a shot of espresso may seem extra tempting to those with fatigue, many doctors actually recommend that people living with fibromyalgia limit their caffeine intake. Coffee and caffeine in general can make it harder to get a good night's sleep, which may make symptoms of fatigue worse.

Also, try to avoid foods that are highly processed, full of refined sugar, fried, or found in a vending machine. This may sound obvious but, generally speaking, these foods tend to be high in saturated and trans fats, carbohydrates and sodium. While they will deliver a quick burst of energy, they will ultimately lead to a crash that will just worsen fatigue and tiredness. These foods also offer little in the way of nutrition and are full of calories, which can lead to weight gain. Carrying extra weight can worsen fibromyalgia pain and lethargy, too.

Avoid Gluten and Limit Dairy
People living with fibromyalgia may be more prone to a gluten sensitivity. Gluten, a protein in wheat and some

other grains, is often present in foods like bread, pasta and crackers, but is also a component of many food ingredients, including thickeners for some ice creams and salad dressings. It's very important to read ingredient labels if you're avoiding gluten in your diet.

Similar to gluten, people with fibromyalgia may be more likely to develop a lactose intolerance, or sensitivity to the natural sugar in dairy products. Remember, however, that low-fat dairy can be an important part of a healthy diet. Not all dairy products may cause symptoms or upset your stomach. Certain foods, such as yogurt, are often tolerated better by those with a lactose intolerance.

Keep an Eye on Additives
Some food additives can act as triggers for people with fibromyalgia, so beware of ingredients like monosodium glutamate (MSG), which is often used in processed foods, fast food and Chinese food, Watch out for certain artificial sweeteners, such as aspartame, too. MSG has been known to cause headaches in some individuals, and

artificial sweeteners can trigger IBS symptoms, including stomach cramps and diarrhea.

A study published in Clinical and Experimental Rheumatology found that MSG may exacerbate fibromyalgia symptoms in some patients. In a four-week study, 37 fibromyalgia patients (all of them had also been diagnosed with IBS) ate an MSG- and aspartame-free diet. At the end of the month, 84 percent of participants reported that their symptoms had improved.

Say No to Nightshades
Overall, the more veggies you eat, the better, if you're living with fibromyalgia. However, one group of vegetables, the nightshade family, seems to irritate some people with the chronic pain condition. If this is the case for you, limit your intake of these veggies-eggplant, potatoes and tomatoes are among the nightshade family members-but don't forget to compensate with other vegetables, as they're nutrient-dense and full of important antioxidants.

How to Create a Fibromyalgia Diet That's Right for You

As far as a fibromyalgia diet goes, one of the best things you can do is keep a food diary. It's difficult to remember and keep track of everything you eat in a day-let alone a week or month-to detect patterns of potentially problematic foods. Having a diet history written down will be a helpful tool for you and a dietitian if you decide to consult one. The diary can help you two detect trends, find out which foods are bothersome and which foods don't cause any issues.

Under a dietitian's supervision, you may want to experiment with eliminating a certain food or a food group you suspect may be a trigger. Most dietitians recommend eliminating these foods or groups of food for a few weeks to see if there's a noticeable difference in how you feel and what you experience when you eat.

The Bottom Line: Though there is no one medical cure or healing diet to alleviate fibromyalgia pain currently, taking a closer look at your food choices, ideally with a registered dietitian, and making some adjustments may help improve symptoms--and lead to a healthier diet and lifestyle overall.

Fibro-Friendly Snack Recipes
Here are a few ways that snacks can be a part of a comprehensive healthy meal plan:

- You're out running errands and won't be home at a regular meal-time.
- You're not very hungry and would prefer a snack to a full meal.
- You need to pack snacks for work or school.
- You need to pack snacks for you or your family while out at sporting events.
- You need snack ideas for camping, family picnics, or outings at the beach.
- You have a high metabolism and need snack ideas for a mid-afternoon boost.

- You don't have time for a meal and need to grab something quickly.

The following ideas are sure to get your creative juices flowing!

Quick & Easy Snacks

Hardboiled Eggs: Eat plain with a little sea salt, or try adding a dash of paprika or a spoonful of guacamole.

Nuts: Raw, when possible – choose almonds, walnuts, macadamias, cashews, Brazil nuts, pistachios, etc.

Seeds: Raw, when possible – try sunflower, pepitas (pumpkin), chia, hemp, ground flax, etc.

Crudités and Handy Veggies: Carrots, celery, cucumbers, jicama, snap peas, peppers cut into strips, broccoli, cauliflower, cherry tomatoes, zucchini, yellow squash, etc.

Fruits: Apples, pears, peaches, oranges, tangerines, grapes, melons, strawberries, raspberries, blackberries, blueberries, cherries, kiwi, etc.

Frozen Fruit Treats: Try frozen grapes, blueberries, sliced strawberries, raspberries, blackberries, cherries, peach chunks, mango chunks, etc. Eat them as is, or add to salads, smoothies, or nut mixes.

Olives: Look for varieties with as few ingredients as possible. The healthy fats in olives can help you to feel sustained energy as well as feeling fuller, longer.

Pickles: Choose homemade varieties or those with natural and recognizable ingredients.

Tuna or Sardines: Canned or packaged – read the label for wild-caught and environmentally-friendly varieties

Veggie, Lentil, or Bean Soups: By the cup or thermos, why not?

"Energy" Bars: If you need a grab-and-go bar, choose a healthy packaged variety such as Kind bars or GoodOnYa Bars, etc. (Better yet, see options below to make your own!)

Simple Combo Snacks
Kale Chips: Drizzle shredded kale with Healthy Oil and bake until crisp. Season as desired.

Cucumbers: Slice as desired and add sea salt, and a few sprinkles of apple cider vinegar (adjust to taste). Garnish with fresh mint if available.

Apples/Pears: Select crisp varieties, slice and top with almond butter, sunflower seeds, grapes, raisins, etc.

Apples/Pears: Slice any variety and drizzle with raw, organic honey (or coconut cream) and a dusting of cinnamon.

Healthy Wraps: Choose options such as coconut or egg wraps – you can also use large leaf greens as wraps such as leaf lettuce, cabbage, Swiss chard, kale, etc. Try spreading hummus, avocado, or salsa on the wrap and then add your favorite greens, sprouts, veggies, beans, or meats. Roll up and enjoy! Don't be afraid to roll up fruits as well into healthy wraps. Fruits go well with avocado.

Almond Butter: (Or cashew butter, or other healthy nut butters.) Lip-smacking good right off the spoon, or you can add sunflower seeds, chia seeds, shredded coconut, raw organic honey, raw cacao nibs, protein powder, etc.

Almond Butter: Spread on crudités such as celery, jicama, or cucumbers. Top with seeds or dried fruits if desired.

Veggies and Hummus: Dip sliced or shredded veggies in creamy hummus for a crunchy/creamy treat.

Fresh Fruit: Cut into bite-sized pieces and skewer onto kabobs for easy handling. Kid-friendly. Makes a fun snack and can be dusted with cinnamon if desired.

Avocado: One of the most versatile snacks there is! Cut in half and serve any of the following ingredients right on top. Try these sweet ingredients: shredded unsweetened coconut, chopped nuts, dollop of almond butter, coconut oil, chopped fruits, cinnamon, scoop of protein powder, etc. Or try these savory ingredients: salsa, fried or poached egg, tuna, shredded veggies, chicken, salmon, etc.

Avocado: Make into Guacamole to use as a spread, a dip, or a topping. Mash ripe avocados with any of the following – salsa, chopped onions (try grilling them first for a unique flavor burst!), cilantro, lemon or lime juice, sea salt, garlic salt, or your ingredient of choice, etc.

Roasted Nuts: Bake on a shallow pan in a 250 degree oven. Or use a dry saucepan over medium heat. Stir often to prevent burning. Roast your favorite nut varieties and sprinkle with cinnamon or desired spice such as cayenne.

Roasted Seeds: Choose sunflower seeds or pepitas, etc. Cook as above for nuts.

Roasted Broccoli or Brussels Sprouts: Cut into bite-sized pieces, drizzle in Healthy Oil, roast in 350 degree oven for about 15-20 minutes until edges become slightly browned. Season as desired.

Freeze Dried Fruits: Select varieties with no added chemicals or sugars. Add to nuts, seeds, shredded coconut, etc. to make your own trail mix

Fruit and Veggie Smoothies: Use natural unsweetened coconut milk or almond milk (or coconut water) and blend with any of the following – protein powders, almond butter, raw cacao powder, cinnamon, nuts, frozen berries, leafy greens, ice if desired. A great pick-me-up!

Turkey or Sliced Meats: Great as the basis for roll ups. Use natural, nitrate-free varieties, spread with guacamole or hummus and add any of the following — spinach leaves, shredded veggies, cooked black beans, garbanzo beans, white beans, fresh herbs such as cilantro, basil, or your fillings of choice.

Fruit and Nut Bowl: Pour coconut or almond milk over favorite nuts, berries, shredded coconut, etc. and favorite spices.

Energy Protein Bars: Try your hand at making your own tasty varieties. With a wealth of options to choose from, there's certainly something that suits your personal dietary needs. Try this Protein Bar Recipe Site for some great ideas.

Faux-Nut Snack

These nutty-tasting beans are simple to make and fun to serve as a snack or party appetizer. They also pack well for lunches and are actually, nut-free.

Ingredients:

- 1 can Garbanzo Beans (a.k.a. chickpeas) – about 15 oz.
- Healthy Oil
- Seasonings of your choice

Directions:

I don't typically recommend canned foods, but I've been able to find canned organic garbanzo beans with no added preservatives, etc. Simply choose the best quality product you can find and rinse very well. Of course, cooking your own beans is fine, too. Pat the rinsed beans dry with a paper towel and remove as much moisture (and "skins" as possible).

Place the beans on a baking tray lined with foil and drizzle with oil. Toss to coat well (go ahead and use your hands!) and roast in a 350 degree oven for about 30 minutes.

Stir every 10 minutes or so and check often. These can burn quickly.

When cooled enough to taste, try one to see if it's still too moist in the middle. If so, return to the oven. Keep testing every 5 minutes or so until done.

Flavor with your favorite seasonings and spices. Go ahead and experiment with sea salt, pepper, dried basil, oregano, thyme, rosemary, chili powder, cayenne, onion powder, garlic powder, etc. From simple sea salt to spices with a bit more kick, there are plenty of options to choose from. If nut allergies aren't a concern, you can add nuts, too, for a great texture combination.

Made in the USA
Columbia, SC
07 November 2023